Where Did She Go?

Experiences of an Alzheimer's Caregiver

Donald A. Noffsinger

Author of *FORWARD EVER!*
and
What is ETERNITY?

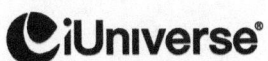

WHERE DID SHE GO?
EXPERIENCES OF AN ALZHEIMER'S CAREGIVER

iUniverse books may be ordered through booksellers or by contacting:

iUniverse
1663 Liberty Drive
Bloomington, IN 47403
www.iuniverse.com
1-800-Authors (1-800-288-4677)

ISBN: 978-1-4917-7267-6 (sc)
ISBN: 978-1-4917-7268-3 (e)

Library of Congress Control Number: 2015913343

Print information available on the last page.

iUniverse rev. date: 09/09/2015

Cover Picture titled "COME WINTER"
painted by Birdie Noffsinger in her early stages of Alzheimer's Disease
Owned by Donald A. Noffsinger
Used by permission.

Scripture quotations marked NIV are taken from the Holy Bible, New International Version®. NIV®. Copyright © 1973, 1978, 1984 by International Bible Society. Used by permission of Zondervan. All rights reserved. [Biblica]

To my four sons, Greg, Ron, Randy, and Mark,
who have brought so much joy
and inspiration to my life!

Contents

Preface

What feelings do you experience when you find that your spouse has physical problems along with mental problems and failing memory? You are disheartened to see that your spouse can no longer take care of him- or herself, cook, do laundry, do the grocery shopping, wash dishes, clean the house, remember where things are in the kitchen, or do or remember all the many other things that go on every day around the normal household. From my perspective, it is harder for a man than it is for a woman who is left in the same position of caring for a husband. But on the other hand, many of the feelings are the same, whichever sex you are.

The feelings that come upon you can take a wide range. Included in the first reactions are those of feeling sorry for yourself. Why do I need to change my whole lifestyle? Why do I have to turn down social invitations for dinners and parties? Why can we no longer take trips to places we've wanted to go? How can I keep my job going and still take care of my spouse and all the household duties? How do I tell others of my wife's or husband's problems? How do I explain my wife's or husband's failing memory? How do I react when I find incorrect answers being given to questions that other people may ask? What am I going to do as the disease progresses to more serious stages? Why, God, does my spouse have to go through this? It isn't fair. Why, God, do I have to change my lifestyle to become a caregiver? How many sacrifices do I have to make?

But soon you find your feelings going in the other direction. How can I help my spouse? How can I make his or her life better? What doctors do I need to find to help in this situation? Are there remedies to help him or her feel better or to delay the progress of Alzheimer's? What can I learn on the Internet that may help me to better understand what his or her problems are all about? What can I learn about my many new roles as a caregiver? Are there books that will help me? Surely others have trodden this path before me and have left tracks for me to follow as I struggle with my new life challenges.

This book is simply part of my personal story of what it feels like to be a full-time caregiver, how I learned to cope, and the sources of help I found along the way. In other words, this book is kind of a road map that may help you in your situation.

For me, the biggest help of all was my personal faith in Jesus Christ, in His love and unfailing promises that held me up when I was ready to fall, and the realization that this life is only temporary, at best— that I am really a citizen of heaven doing temporary duty here on earth. So, along the way in this book, I will be encouraging you to trust in God, pray often, read your Bible, study good Christian resources, and find your own spiritual footholds to help you and your spirit remain strong along your path as a caregiver.

Chapter 1

Dementia

Dementia is a devastating disease.

It is devastating both for the person with the mental decline and also for the husband (or wife) who has to stand by as the helper, while feeling helpless as the downhill slide progresses. In my case, my wife had a brilliant mind. She was trained as a nurse and also had a degree in art. She loved being a mother and a homemaker, loved to travel, was a very active church teacher and leader, and was an independent person. But now she was more like a two-year-old.

The big difference is that if you have a two-year-old child, you take pride each day in seeing the progress he or she is making in learning new words, the names of new people, how to walk or run better, or how to get dressed. What I saw was my wife losing words and forgetting the names of close friends (and even family members); her vocabulary was losing more words each day. She was stumbling more as she walked, couldn't find food or utensils in her own kitchen, and could no longer get dressed by herself.

So instead of seeing the two-year-old make progress each day and become more independent, with dementia you watch the slippery slope downward toward complete dependence on you to supply your spouse's daily needs.

In many ways it may be harder for the caregiver husband (or wife) than it is for the person with the disease. My wife used to be more nervous, more concerned about a lot of things, more worried about her looks and all those many things, but now her worries were next to none; in fact, her mind became more of a blank each day. So just as a two-year-old has few worries, so also is the state of mind of a person with dementia as the disease progresses to the more severe stages. As part of that progression, you, as the caregiver, lose the companionship of your lifelong mate—and the blessing the two of you have developed over the years to share your many joys and sorrows and to learn from each other's perspectives on life.

From a man's perspective, I believe it is much easier for a woman to be the caregiver, since she has already spent many years caring for young children, taking care of a house, cooking, and so forth, while the man has been outside the home, trying to make a living for the family. (Sound like a chauvinist male's opinion?)

How do you cope? For the person with dementia, he or she simply relaxes and depends more and more on the caregiver to supply the needed food, clothing, bedding, and the like, for each day. But for the caregiver, the opposite is true. You, as caregiver, start to worry more and more about where the future is leading. How can I learn all the many new skills required to cope with my husband's or wife's increasing needs? Where does the future lead? Can I handle it? When is it time for a nursing home to take over? Where do I go for help? What about the financial side of life? Will I wind up broke? What about my own well-being—the lack of social life, increasingly being tied to home, losing contact with friends and the outside world, feeling lonely, feeling forgotten, and all the many other elements that start to take over your thinking hours?

That's what this book is all about: sharing with you the helpful things I have learned during the years as my wife's dementia went from mild to moderate to moderately severe and then to the severe stage—ending in death. It is not an easy journey, but it can be a rewarding journey in learning more about what life is all about. Without my deep Christian faith, it would have been a much harder (or even impossible) journey for me. But Christ has been by my side each day, calming my fears, giving new insights, increasing my faith in the future, and giving me hope in realizing more and more how temporary this life is anyway— and that He is giving each of us a chance, through caring for others, to understand better His message that saves our souls from so many earthly worries and concerns. He is also helping us understand how to trust more fully in His guidance to meet the needs of each day. As the Bible says in Psalm 56:3–4, "When

I am afraid, I will trust in you, in God, whose word is praise, I will not be afraid".

So come with me as we look at the various aspects of your new job as caregiver, such as how to cope. But more than that, we will look at some of the plentiful help offered in the book of books, the Bible, for the wisdom needed in your new caregiving tasks, along with help in choosing your own attitude and the thoughts you will allow to occupy your mind as you face the various challenges of each new day.

Here is a psalm I found very helpful in calming my fears of how I would be able to handle all the daunting tasks that were coming each day. This is how David felt when he was desperate and overwhelmed as he was being pursued by Saul and was hiding away in a cave:

Psalm 142

I cry aloud to the Lord;
I lift up my voice to the Lord for mercy.
I pour out my complaints before Him;
Before him I tell my troubles.
When my spirit grows faint within me,
It is You who knows my way.
In the path where I walk
Men have laid a snare for me.
Look to my right and see
No one is concerned for me.
I have no refuge
No one cares for my life

I cry to you, O LORD:
I say "You are my refuge,
My portion in the land of the living."
Listen to my cry:
For I am in desperate need
Rescue me from those who pursue me,
For they are too strong for me.
Set me free from my prison,
That I may praise your name.
Then the righteous will gather
around me,
Because of your goodness to me!

Did you note how close David was to giving up? But then he remembers God's promises to listen to his cry for help. I believe He gives the same invitation and promises to you and me. Remind yourself of His promise in Matthew 11:28–29, where He says, "Take my yoke upon you and learn from Me, for I am gentle and humble in heart, and you will find rest for your souls."

In every difficult situation
is potential value
Believe this
Then begin looking for it!

—Norman Vincent Peale

Chapter 2

Payback Time

"Payback time" is a phrase used by one of my friends whose wife had Alzheimer's. When I first heard him using the term, my reactions were not positive. I think I felt that the term was too strong, since each mate carries his or her own share of the burdens in raising a family, taking care of a home, fulfilling social obligations, and so forth. But as time progressed, I found myself thinking more and more about that phrase as I was doing everything around the house—all the shopping, all the cooking, and all those mundane chores.

While I still feel that each of us carried our own share of the load in raising our family, I came to realize more and more how tied up I was in an occupation I loved, and beyond that I spent many evening hours in civic activities, board meetings, church duties, and all those good things while Birdie was left home alone to "keep things going." Yes, all my activities helped us keep bread on the table and provide for our four growing sons, but I now realize how much I owe to her for holding things together at home while I was running around the city, taking business trips all over the country, even a trip to Europe, and so forth. So my mind finally "softened" enough to realize that perhaps this was payback time.

It is easy for all of us to feel like martyrs, feel like we are carrying more than 50 percent of the load or "giving in" more than half the time on disagreements that come in our marriages. I certainly felt that way many times—that I was the one out there making enough money to keep the family going financially and yet my wife expected me to do all the many things on the "honey-do" lists she always had. And when invitations came to play golf on a Saturday, she put her foot down and said I needed to be home at least once in a while to help with things that needed done. And on top of that, she had developed her own way of doing things, so when I did try to help, my own way of approaching problems was not always pleasing to her. Sound familiar in your own situation?

For a man, it takes a lot of adjustments to finally "slow down" and come to the place in which you find fulfillment in being the full-time caregiver for your wife with dementia (or Alzheimer's). There are many dimensions to the new routine:

a. Suddenly I was the "boss" around home. Everything got done my way because she had forgotten how to do anything.
b. She depended on me for nearly everything, like a two-year-old child.

c. I became more appreciative of the disagreements we'd had along the way, and came to realize the wisdom she'd had in many things and how she helped me so much in learning how to live life.

d. Seeing your wife die a slow death makes you think more about life, about what is truly important, about the values of family, and about eternal life as promised to us as believers in Christ.

e. It forces you to think more about all the blessings the Lord has bestowed upon you during life and each day, and to think less about all your current problems.

The Bible has many aids for us to think about as we walk this road of being the caregiver for our spouses with Alzheimer's. One scripture that often comes to mind is a favorite for many people—Psalm 23:

> The Lord is my shepherd
> I shall not be in want
> He makes me to lie down
> In green pastures
> He leads me beside quiet waters
> He restores my soul
> He leads me in paths of righteousness
> For His name's sake
> Even though I walk through the valley
> Of the shadow of death
> I will fear no evil
> For you are with me

Your rod and your staff
They comfort me
You prepare a table before me
In the presence of my enemies
You anoint my head with oil
My cup overflows
Surely goodness and love will follow me
All the days of my life
And I will dwell in the house of the Lord
Forever!

Or, when feeling a bit low, I found it helpful to let my mind run over the tune and words of the old Christian hymn, "Count Your Blessings." The words of the first verse are especially appropriate when you are feeling the full load of all your cares and worries about where the future will lead. Here are the words:

Verse 1
When upon life's billows you are tempest tossed,
When you are discouraged thinking all is lost,
Count your many blessings, name them one by one,
And it will surprise you what the Lord has done!

Verse 2
Are you ever burdened with a load of care?

Does the cross seem heavy you are called
to bear?
Count your many blessings, every doubt
will fly,
And you will be singing as the days go by!

Verse 3
When you look at others with their land
a gold,
Think that Christ has promised you his
wealth untold,
Count your many blessings; money
cannot buy,
Your reward in heaven, nor your one on
high.

Verse 4
So, amid the conflict, whether great or
small,
Do not be discouraged, God is over all.
Count your many blessings, angels will
attend,
Help and comfort give you, to your
journey's end.

Refrain
Count your many blessings, name them
one by one.
Count your many blessings, see what God
hath done!

It is best to learn wisdom through
the experience of others!

—Latin Proverb

Chapter 3

Analyze This

One of my strong points in business management was my ability to analyze situations—and come up with good solutions to fix the problem. So I figured that I would try that ability on this situation to see if I could come up with a solution to "fix" my wife's growing problems. Here is some of what I did in this endeavor.

I started out with a review of my wife's history and the things that may have affected her in her journey of life. I wanted to see if there were things in her background that may have contributed to the mental problems and paranoia that preceded the onset of Alzheimer's disease.

When I first met Birdie in 1954, she was a twenty-five-year-old widow with three small children. I first noticed her when I was singing in the church choir in Defiance, Ohio, and noted this beautiful new lady in the audience. It was hard to miss her since she was holding a young child and swaying back and forth to keep the child quiet. Beside her were two other young children, but no husband did I see. During the following weeks, I made inquiries about this lady and found out that she had just lost her husband to cancer and that she had moved from Chicago back to Defiance to be near her in-laws, who attended my church. Her family lived in California, but she had lived in Defiance before and had decided to move back there again.

So this was a big change and adjustment in her life. Her husband had been a promising young executive. His company had sent him to Boston for a one-year executive development course at MIT, and they had just moved back to Chicago. Just a month after the move back to Chicago, he had developed cancer—a fast moving cancer—and died less than three months later. So this was a big blow in her life. (In the midst of all this change, her father died in 1954, and her mother died in 1956.)

I started chatting with her, and then invited her to join me at the church's singles fellowship group meetings. I found her to be a very good mother to her three sons and a real "trooper" with strong stamina, strong Christian faith, and a faith in the future that made her determined not to give up on life but rather to proceed with faith. We were married in the spring of 1955.

A year later, she delivered our fourth son, Mark. But a year after that, the next pregnancy turned into a tubal pregnancy, requiring emergency surgery. It resulted in the loss of the child and a serious struggle for recovery by Birdie. This I would say was another big trauma in her life, both physically and mentally, since we had planned to have two more children for a family total of eight.

(Think how much her life changed in just four short years: she moved from Boston to Chicago, her husband died, she moved to Defiance, her father died, she married a new husband, she had another child, her mother died, and then she had a tubal pregnancy. All of these life-changing events, so close together, took a toll on her life.)

A complete hysterectomy in 1963 seemed to be another trauma for her. It seemed to affect her nervous system and brought changes in her entire personality. She became a much tenser person. She became less open and felt that people were talking about her and plotting against her—all signs of paranoia setting in. And about this time she developed type 2 diabetes. All together, these things had effects on her physical body, which brought on more major surgeries.

In spite of all of the above, she had some good years. She worked as a nurse in a local hospital for seven years and then went back to college to earn a degree in art. Then she became the art gallery director for Anderson University. She resigned from that position in 1975 so she could travel with me to many places around the world in my new position as president of Warner Press, Inc.

But during those years the paranoia increased, and she endured more major surgeries. She endured a thyroidectomy, the removal of her gall bladder, and back surgery. She also suffered broken wrists from falls. The list goes on and on. Did all of these traumatic events contribute to the dementia and the onset of Alzheimer's? There is no proof that it did, though as you can guess, in my mind the answer is yes. It must have played a part in the whole process.

It was hard on me to "keep things going" during so many surgeries, but the hardest part for me was the progression of her paranoia. As is so often the case, the brunt of the distrust and accusations falls on the person or persons closest to them. So I, as her husband, was the usual target. These were very difficult years for me. The worst accusation came when she accused me of having an affair with one of our daughters-in-law. This daughter-in-law had been one of her favorites, so she got the accusation too. The big blowup came when our son and daughter-in-law were visiting with us and my wife told them they were no longer welcome in our home. In that evening's blowup, she became very distraught emotionally, which seemed to me like a complete nervous and mental breakdown. This was the first revelation to the family of the problems she was having. This was in 1999. With the mental problems now out in the open, and with the help of our son Mark, who was a doctor, we were able to get her admitted to a mental hospital in Grand Rapids, Michigan, for several weeks' treatment. After that she became somewhat better again, but she still had relapses.

The more rapid decline, both physically and mentally, came after a series of four major surgeries for bowel problems and carotid artery problems during the year 2003. Then with the dementia problems progressing, she fell in early 2005 and broke her shoulder. Later that same year, she fell again and broke the other shoulder. Mentally and physically, the downhill slide progressed each day.

This short recap of the first fifty years of our marriage will give you some perspective on the things I had learned up to this point—and that I knew something about caregiving—but little did I know the even bigger challenges that the next few years held in store.

My training in business was to analyze the problem and then fix it. One of my solutions was a change of neighborhood. Birdie had become paranoid about our neighbors, and maybe a whole new set of neighbors would be the solution to the paranoia problems. So we moved across town. It helped for a while, but then the same old problems developed. Later I felt that a complete change of location could help the problem, since we had been involved in so much church politics in my role as president of the church publishing house. So after my retirement, we moved to Kalamazoo, Michigan, to be near our son and family. For a while this seemed to help, but soon the paranoia resumed as usual. So my attempts to fix things by moving did not pan out as far as her paranoia was concerned.

And as I learned later, it is not unusual for people with Alzheimer's to suffer through paranoia problems before the onset of dementia problems. So in my wife's case, you could say that all the signals were showing up, but I was slow in recognizing all the symptoms because her doctor never even mentioned dementia to me. The first I heard of the diagnosis was on a written report the doctor had prepared on her situation. Later he did prescribe medications like Aricept and Namenda, which may have slowed the progress of the disease, but in general my feeling was that the doctor was very well trained in physical problems but did not want to get involved in mental problems.

The net result of all this analysis was the realization that I couldn't fix it. That is a frustrating conclusion to accept for a man who is used to fixing things. So my role was to stop analyzing and instead use all my energies to give care.

We are still masters of our fate
We are still captains of our souls!

—Winston Churchill

Chapter 4

What Are My Duties as Caregiver?

Early on in the caregiving process, after I moved my office home so I could be with my wife throughout the day, I sat one day and thought to myself, *What is this job all about?* My life had changed so much. My wife had always been the home manager. She had taken care of nearly everything around the house, and suddenly there I was in charge of everything—the cooking, the laundry, the housecleaning, the grocery buying, the bed making, the outside work, and so on. In fact, if anything happened around the house, it was up to *me*! Now that was quite a revelation in thinking about the change that had taken place!

So, being the lifetime analyst and business thinker that I have always been and having written many, many position descriptions to help other people understand their jobs in the business world, I set about writing a position description for myself. This exercise helped me see more clearly where I was headed, and it served as a reference point as additional changes arose with the progression of my wife's Alzheimer's disease.

Here is the "position description" I wrote for myself that day:

Caregiver Manager
Duties, Responsibilities, and Privileges

> If I am not for myself, who will ever be for me?
> If I am only for myself, what am I?
> And if not now, when?
> —*Quote from a Jewish sage who lived at
> the time of Jesus. (Timeless words!)*

The above "wisdom" indicates that if I do not take care of Donald, who will? On the other hand, if all I care about is Donald, of what value am I?

The average "caregiver" lasts about four years and then heads downhill to the level of the care receiver. To avoid that rapid decline, I must find ways to take care of Donald as Birdie's dementia goes downhill. How do I do that?

1. Think of myself as the *caregiver manager* and not just as the only caregiver Birdie has. There are many helpers around that I need to get involved in our lives in the years ahead. I need to think of myself in the same way I think of the property manager for Cannaan Properties or the president of Warner Press, all the while employing the necessary talents to get the caregiving jobs done in the best way and with love and appreciation for Birdie for all the good

years we have enjoyed together and for all she has done for me over the past fifty years!

2. How do I implement the above philosophy?

    a. Hire a housekeeper for at least one day per week to clean the house and to be here for Birdie on that day. If possible, it should be for Thursday, my golf day. I could even play eighteen holes again!

    b. Don't allow the stress of caregiving to get to me. If I see that happening, I need to arrange for the necessary help so I can take a respite, a weekend away, or a golfing trip, or whatever to regain perspective.

    c. Educate myself in the nature of Alzheimer's disease by attending Alzheimer's caregiver group meetings to make new acquaintances and learn from the experiences of other caregivers in how they cope with the problems. Such meetings will also help me to better know the resources available in the Kalamazoo community.

    d. Write down all of Birdie's medicines, keep a record of all the comments from the medical professionals, and have benchmarks to refer to as progress up or down is noted.

    e. Hold a family conference to review the plans that are being made for Birdie's ongoing care.

    f. Research services available in the Kalamazoo area for adult day care, nursing facilities, volunteer programs, church programs, and so on. Look at them in two ways: how they will help Birdie and how they might help me.

g. Be a part of a support group, to gain both ideas for Birdie's care and friendship for me.

h. Make sure that all of Birdie's documents are up-to-date (living will, etc.) as well as her lists of desires that she previously prepared for disposition of jewelry, et cetera.

i. Be willing to tell others that I need help and learn to accept their help. Don't be too proud to acknowledge my need for help.

j. Approach some of the hardest caregiving tasks as a professional and not one so deeply emotionally involved as I am. Step back at times to look at the situation as a professional. Consider all of the practical aspects. Don't let myself get buried in my emotional concerns.

k. Financial planning is required to make certain that we can afford all of the above suggested aids and to determine for how long. Check out other resources that might be available, such as Medicare for home care, and so on.

3. Prepare a detailed medical information form that lists all of the known facts about Birdie's situation and then review the information with her primary care physician and/or other medical professionals to help in their diagnoses and help me know how to handle various situations that might arise.

4. Help Birdie to have a life of hope and meaning to whatever extent possible.

5. Learn how to handle my own grief in no longer being able to travel, not getting trips to see our kids or sister or friends, Birdie not going to church with me, not attending Bunco or other parties to have fellowship with friends, feeling shut off and shut up from the world, no longer having the office to go to each day away from home, all of those many elements of the missing parts of life, along with the lack of companionship (in a normal way) with Birdie.

6. Make a list of all of my various worries about the future and then realize that I can only live one day at a time! Study the Bible for insights on life, and look to the long range future of life eternal with Christ.

7. Keep the family informed on Birdie's progress.

This position description was a great help to me. It helped me keep my mind on the overall goal of giving my wife the best care I knew how to give, and it also encouraged me to involve other people's necessary talents as the needs arose.

The next several chapters of this book will give more details on what I learned along the way as I dealt with many of the duties, responsibilities, and privileges of being a caregiver.

God is our refuge and strength,
an ever present help in trouble!

—Psalm 46:1

Chapter 5

Educate Yourself

One of the steps in the position description I wrote for myself as caregiver manager was to educate myself about the nature of Alzheimer's disease.

In following this assignment to myself, I found it quite helpful to learn from the experiences of others and to have a much better grasp on what to expect as each new stage of the disease presented itself in my wife's situation.

The Internet

One of the first places I turned to was the Internet. When you use the Google search engine for the words *dementia* or *Alzheimer's*, it comes up with pages of websites that offer various viewpoints about many aspects of this devastating disease. One of the most helpful websites is the one sponsored by the Alzheimer's Association, www.alz.org.

Within this website, the Alzheimer's Association has a section called "Your Personal Carefinder," and one of the resources within that section is a questionnaire to help you ascertain what stage of the disease your care receiver is in. It asks questions about your care receiver's abilities, including the following:

a. Responsibility for his or her own medications
b. Independent planning, preparing, and serving of meals
c. Modes of transportation (meaning can he or she still drive or use public transportation)
d. Independent planning and completion of laundry
e. Ability to maintain house alone or with what degrees of assistance
f. Ability to handle finances
g. Ability to handle shopping needs
h. Ability to use the telephone
i. Ability to eat without assistance

I found answering these questions to be quite helpful in realizing how far my wife had slipped in her routine abilities to handle things around the house. It's amazing how things that at one time took no thought at all for her to do were now beyond her capabilities. For a husband, it was a sad process to watch unfold.

After you complete the questionnaire, the Alzheimer's website then lists the characteristics of the seven stages of the disease. From these charts, you can then ascertain the status of your care receiver, helping you to know what stage of the diseases he or she is now in.

The website then recommends care options for your consideration, and if outside help is recommended, it gives you a list of questions you should ask potential helpers as you choose among the many options available to you (home care, day care, assisted living, nursing homes, etc.).

You will also find many other websites that give helpful information, and all you need to do is use a search engine like Google to search for Alzheimer's disease. References galore will come up on your screen.

Talking with Others

Whenever the opportunity presented itself, I found it most helpful to talk with other caregivers who were facing the same problems as me. Many of them were several steps ahead of me, while others were several steps behind me (meaning their spouses were several steps behind the stage my wife had reached at that time) and I was able to help them. For me, these opportunities came mainly whenever I had the chance to attend a seminar or meeting regarding Alzheimer's, and I would then have the opportunity to chat with the other attendees. I found that I learned a lot and gained the knowledge that I was not alone in being a lonely caregiver. I was one of many in my community struggling with the same caregiving problems.

Printed Materials

Books, pamphlets, and other printed materials of all kinds are readily available—good materials that deal with the many aspects of Alzheimer's disease, the history of it, the lack of solutions to it, and how to cope with caregiving problems. I found many of these printed resources to be quite helpful, but the main thing you learn is that so far there is no cure. You can be the best caregiver in the whole wide world, but your spouse will still face a future of going downhill until death comes as the final resolution of the problem. That was my fatalistic viewpoint of the whole matter. But in the meantime, you have to learn all you can to deal with the daily situations you face.

(I should be more careful about what I am writing. This is one of those printed materials, but this is the type of book I wish I had found when I was struggling as a caregiver!)

Television Programs
Another good source of learning is to watch special television programs dealing with Alzheimer's disease. Some of these programs are very well done, and all you have to do is sit and watch!

As I was with Moses,
So I will be with you.
I will not leave you nor forsake you.
Be strong and courageous!

—Joshua 1:5–6

Chapter 6

A Life of Hope and Meaning

Item 4 in the caregiver manager position description says to *help Birdie to have a life of hope and meaning to whatever extent possible.* How can you or I as the caregiving spouse accomplish such a high goal?

I have found that there are many facets and different approaches to helping your spouse have a more satisfying life in spite of his or her memory problems. Here a few examples of what I have found:

1. Limit his or her number of choices. For example, when going to a restaurant I found that the number of choices offered in the menu was overwhelming to her. Since I knew what kinds of food she liked in the past, I tried to narrow it down to one or two items that might sound good to her at the time. But often it wound up that she would have the same thing I chose, and that turned out to be a pretty good route since her appetite had diminished. So often my solution was to order a full-sized meal to be split between the two of us. That way she could eat all she wanted and I usually had a more than sufficient

portion left for me. And she was saved from the confusion of trying to make a decision and of having a lot of leftover food. At home, I stopped asking her what she would like to have for meals because that was confusing for her to answer. So, as "chief cook," I proceeded with whatever menu came to mind, and she was usually quite happy to have the decision made for her.

2. Stop correcting his or her incorrect answers or statements. I was guilty of constantly trying to correct what she was telling me or others about various events or family information. It was hard for me to learn to simply let it pass and then to give the correct information only if the person she was talking to asked questions. When just the two of us were talking, I might ask her if that was the way she saw it. But correcting her made her frustrated, and then she would try even harder to convince me that her statements were correct. It was a losing battle for me and a big frustration for her.

3. Lower your expectations. As my wife's disease progressed, I found that as caregiver I needed to constantly lower my expectations of what she could do. Even something as simple as helping set the table for a meal at times was beyond her capabilities. She needed help choosing silverware and then couldn't remember how to place it around the plates. But again, rather than criticize, I learned to express my appreciation

to her for the help she was giving, et cetera. You must constantly remember that the brilliant mind your loved one once had has reduced itself to the level of a young child.

4. Express your love for your loved one and build him or her up in any way possible. I found that my wife responded favorably and tended to feel better about herself when I told her how beautiful she was and how much I loved her or if I praised her for doing something well.

5. Sing hymns together. I found several TV church programs with congregations singing the old hymns we enjoyed so much. I found that if I tuned in to one of those programs and then started to sing along with the congregation, she would often join in and try to sing along also.

6. Read the Bible or inspirational stories to your spouse. I noticed that my wife seemed to follow along fairly well when I read to her from the Bible or read inspirational stories from magazines like *Guideposts*.

7. Talk about family and old friends. Even though your spouse might not remember, he or she may enjoy hearing about family events of the past, special times with close friends, or other major life occurrences you have enjoyed together.

8. Be watchful to prevent missteps or falls. As a person's ability to walk diminishes, the likelihood of slipping or falling increases. My wife fell several times, resulting in broken

shoulders and other injuries. So I learned to be much more observant and helpful in order to prevent recurrences of these problems.

9. Use nightlights.
10. Be safety minded at all times.
11. Plan ahead.
12. Keep your own spirits up!

Come to me
All you who are weary and burdened
And I will give you rest!

—Matthew 11:28

Chapter 7

How Am I Doing as Caregiver?

As time went by, I began to wonder how I was doing in this job as caregiver and if Birdie was going downhill or if it was just my imagination. It seemed that her doctor did not have time to deal with her mental decline, other than to say that she had dementia and to prescribe the best-known pills for possibly slowing the progress of Alzheimer's. So where could I go to get a knowledgeable assessment of where we were? It was hard for me to know just how far the disease had progressed, since the downhill slide is so slow and there were days when she was much more "with it." I felt the need for a professional to give me an opinion. And I wanted to know how I might improve my caregiving routines. Was I doing things in the best ways possible? It had been pretty much a "learn to do by doing" routine as the workload increased day by day.

While I was attending one of the workshops sponsored by the Alzheimer's Association, someone recommended that I have a geriatric nurse come to my home for a firsthand review of Birdie's situation. The nurse could also give me practical suggestions that might help in my daily role as caregiver.

On September 25, 2006—a beautiful fall day—the geriatric nurse arrived at our home. She arrived at about nine thirty in the morning and was there until noon.

First on her agenda was to talk with Birdie and to appraise the degree to which the dementia was progressing. She asked various questions to see if Birdie could answer them, tried some simple memory tests, reviewed her medical condition, and tested her ability to respond to or understand what we were talking about. In general, Birdie was cooperative.

She reported to me that Birdie was in the third stage of four; in other words, she was now in the stage of serious dementia. I had not thought it was quite that far along. This appraisal was very helpful to me—having a professional person who did these type of appraisals every day take the time for a far more detailed review than a medical doctor had time for.

In addition to the appraisal, here is a list of some of the very practical advice I received that day, all of which helped relieve the stress of wondering if I was doing the right things:

1. Remove Lifeline. The nurse's recommendation was that I save the expense of the Lifeline I had installed, because Birdie would not know how to use it anyway.

2. Carry a note in my billfold in case I was in an accident so that people would know to send

help to the house for Birdie. The note could be quite simple and say, *I am full-time caregiver for my wife who has dementia. If I am injured, please send help to her: Birdie F. Noffsinger, 7188 Eagle Heights Drive, Mattawan, MI 49071, phone 269-375-3572 (but she will not answer the phone). Also call my son Mark at 269-375-9234.*

3. Do not get a power lift chair for Birdie. The nurse said the mechanism would scare her even if she could learn how to use it.

4. Go to the Alzheimer's Association office to get a supply of cards I could use in restaurants to inform the waitress that my companion has Alzheimer's. While at the office, also get a "safe return" bracelet for Birdie to wear in case she ever wandered out of the house.

5. Consider the use of a baby monitor so that when I was in other areas of the house I could hear anything unusual going on.

6. Talk with her doctor about the hallucinations she was having because he might be able to prescribe something to help.

7. Purchase a lifelike newborn baby at Toys "R" Us for Birdie since she had such a love for babies. She told me that this had worked quite well with other similar dementia cases.

8. Find temporary help. If I wanted to be gone for a day or even a weekend, she told me how to secure temporary nonmedical assistance.

She suggested a local firm called Stay Home Companion that had received good reviews. The price at that time was around eighteen to twenty-five dollars an hour.

9. Start extending my base of support so that when the care needs got beyond my capabilities or endurance, I could get in-home help. However, it is extremely expensive if needed seven days per week or progressed to needing help twenty-four hours per day.

10. Research day care centers. She told me of a Lutheran church that ran a day care center for persons with Alzheimer's. You could take your loved one to stay for a few hours while you took care of errands and other needs. (Note: I did go to inspect the day care center and found it to be a very clean and well-run pleasant place, but I felt that Birdie was already too far along in the disease for me to utilize it for her.)

11. Meet with other caregivers at the Covenant Church each month. In these meetings caregivers exchanged concerns and how-to information. (Note: I attended two of these meetings and found it very helpful to sit down with other caregivers and share our mutual woes and ideas on how to do things. There were only four of us there—three caregiving ladies and one caregiving man (me). But that is usual in this stage of life. I found that in most meetings I

went to the ratio was usually around seven to one—seven women for every man.)

12. Start shopping around for long-term care facilities that take Alzheimer's patients. The nurse told me it was much better to shop around now rather than waiting until it became an urgent situation. For example, if Birdie fell and broke a hip, I would need to find something in a hurry. She suggested several good nursing homes that had special units for dementia patients. Her slogan was "Move ahead of the need. Don't wait 'til it's urgent." She told me Birdie was far enough along to be ready for a facility. She then told me what she knew about four or five such facilities, their lockdown capabilities, the management, whether reports on their caregiving were good or bad, and so forth. This information proved quite helpful to me as I started the shopping process. (I will devote the next chapter to reviewing the steps I took in that process).

13. Review long-term care (LTC) insurance coverage. The nurse was knowledgeable in the terminology of LTC insurance and was pleased to find that Birdie's policy, which we had carried for about twenty years, would provide good financial aid for her caregiving needs.

14. Make sure Birdie's living will was in order. The nurse reviewed Birdie's patient advocate forms and was pleased that Birdie had signed them before she had dementia problems.

15. Visit a geriatric assessment center. The nurse told me of a local hospital that was holding a geriatric assessment center in case I wanted a more thorough review of Birdie's situation, but she informed me the important thing to remember was that the disease would progress and there were no known cures available at that time.

During our discussions that morning, the geriatric nurse was also very helpful in answering many of my questions about my day-to-day caregiving concerns, including the following:

1. Diapers: Since I was a novice at shopping for diapers, she told me I needed to buy the pull-up type with the ruffles. She told me the size to buy and the differences between some of the brands. This information made me a much more confident diaper shopper!

2. Fiber: She said Birdie needed to take Fibercom to give more bulk to her bowel movements and provide some degree of regularity.

3. Hydration: She suggested I use a one-quart pitcher so I would know how much Birdie had drunk during the day. She also said that if Birdie had any urinary problems, I could use cranberry juice.

4. Dental hygiene: The best way to help Birdie brush her teeth was to stand behind her and reach around as if I were doing my own teeth.

5. Appetite: A declining appetite for food is part of Alzheimer's disease. To give Birdie more nourishment, I could try canned supplements like Insure or Boost, starting with a third of a can and working up from there.

6. Bed Sores: Not a problem at that time.

7. Wardrobe: The nurse said to stop using pullover tops and start using button-front type blouses. This would alleviate shoulder pain problems that usually came from the arm motions required when putting on and taking off pullover tops.

8. Bath time: I needed to get a shower attachment with flexible tubing so Birdie could sit on the shower bench and wash herself with the shower wand. This should improve her safety while in the shower.

As you can see from this list of practical advice, I felt it was a very fruitful morning. The visit greatly helped increase my confidence as a caregiver and in where it was all leading.

The billing for the nurse's services was very reasonable for a personal home visit, and it included another visit to my home a few days later to deliver helpful printed materials.

Here is the wording on the invoice I received for the nurse's services:

Initial consultation with Mr. and Mrs. Noffsinger to open file, document health history, address current concerns, offer suggestions for meeting needs due to chronic conditions, consider options for changers as disease process advances, provide support for excellent caregiving already taking place.

Based on this experience, I highly recommend that you seek a consultation with a geriatric nurse to help you develop your road map for the caregiving situation in which you find yourself.

Do not be afraid
Or discouraged.
For the Lord your God is with you
Wherever you go!

—Joshua 1:9

Chapter 8

Shopping for Full-Time Care Facility

In November 2006, I started the daunting task of shopping for what I felt was the right nursing home or assisted-living home for Birdie. The geriatric nurse had told me that I should be doing this, plus I was feeling more worn down from the daily tasks of caregiving.

So the first task was to think about what I was looking for. My list included things like this:

1. Does the place smell good? Here, I was thinking that so many places I had visited had the "nursing home smell" of urine, body odor, and so on. I did not want Birdie to have to live in that atmosphere; neither did I want to visit her in a place like that.

2. Is the staff upbeat in dealing with their patients? Does the staff appear to make it a cheerful place or a downbeat woe-is-me place? Here again, I had seen both and didn't want a place in which every patient was considered a big burden. Rather, I wanted a place that saw each patient as an opportunity for service.

3. Is the place within easy driving distance for me? This was an important question since I was going to be the one making daily trips to visit Birdie.

4. What about the food service? Is the food served in a homey atmosphere or in an institutional kind of way? I was hoping to find a place where the food service was appealing: good food served appropriately.

5. What were the results of their latest inspection by the state? These are listed on the state's website for nursing home inspections. Were there any serious concerns noted?

6. Is a private room available for Birdie? I wanted a private room that was cheery and clean, with a good window view. If so, is it affordable?

7. Is the staff-to-patient ratio less than ten patients per staff person? It should be.

8. Is this a place that will take Birdie through to death? Most of all, that was the kind of place I was looking for. (I already knew of some places that took dementia patients up to a certain level, but then the patient had to move to a different place for more intensive care during the final weeks or months of life.)

Based on the above criteria, I prepared a list of possible sites and began calling for appointments.

Option 1

My first appointment was at a retirement center I had been seriously considering for myself. This very nice facility offered excellent apartments for retirement living. Then, if health needs arose, they had a separate wing devoted to assisted living. Then, if your health needs called for even more care, they had a separate nursing home building that appeared very nice from the outside. So naturally I thought that this would be really ideal. If I moved into the retirement home section, I could just walk next door to visit Birdie each day.

My tour of the nursing home portion was conducted by the community relationships director. But it turned out that the nursing home building smelled like a nursing home and the Alzheimer's wing of the nursing home did not have good lockdown facilities for dementia patients and did not offer private rooms for such patients. Based on these negative points, I quickly decided against this option.

Option 2

The second appointment was at another retirement home with similar facilities for progressive care. In the tour of this facility, I was pleased with the smell, the food service, and the way they had the Alzheimer's patients living in small groups of about twelve, like a family. The lockdown facilities were excellent, the rooms were cheery, the food service very good, and so forth. So it was agreed that we would have their director of admissions for Alzheimer's patients come to our home for a personal review and analysis of Birdie's situation.

On November 6, 2006, the care administrator came to our home. It turned out that the methods used by this RN were very similar to the visit by the geriatric nurse. The first thing on her agenda was to assess Birdie's progress in the stages of Alzheimer's. Following the tests, she stated that Birdie had scored fifty-four points—too many points for admission! She explained that the maximum points for staying in the Alzheimer's section was fifty-eight and that Birdie was already too close to that number to allow admission. After a patient reached fifty-eight points, they had to be be transferred to a higher care facility—to the facility's nursing home or to wherever the family desired—but they could not stay any longer in the facility's Alzheimer's unit.

The nursing home that was part of their complex did not smell good, and I had heard that it had management problems, so this possibility fell to the bottom of my list.

Before the RN left that day, she reviewed my caregiving procedures and felt that I was doing very well. She said it was probably best for Birdie to continue on in my care for several more months if I secured some outside help. But, she stated that if the caregiving tasks were starting to wear me down, it was definitely time for a full-time care facility. So once again, I felt reassured to have another professional opinion on where we were and what I should be doing as caregiver.

Option 3

The next appointment was with the administrator at another facility that looked excellent from the outside, but it was one I had heard some bad publicity about. But I wanted to check it out to see what I thought of it. This was probably the best looking building from the outside, and it was a pleasant place on the inside, with two separate eating rooms—one for those who needed help with food and the other for those who could still feed themselves. The kitchen was adjacent to the two dining rooms. All thirty-four of their patient rooms were private rooms with private baths. The administrator told me that the staff ratio varied according to the degree of needs; they had time studies of all the activities and staff accordingly. She said that presently the overall rate was one staff person per six patients. My impression, though, was that this was a more "commercially run" place, with each patient considered as a unit of work rather than as a person.

I asked her about the bad publicity from a few years ago. Her answer was that the problems had all been resolved. She said they had passed another inspection two weeks ago.

When I asked her how fast Birdie would adjust to facilities like this, her answer was, "She will adjust faster than you will." She said the adjustment time varied but that it was usually fairly fast. Others might take up to thirty days.

All in all, I felt that this was a very nice facility, but somehow the environment just didn't seem as friendly as it should be for a care facility. And I was very possibly influenced by the bad publicity they had gone through.

Option 4

On another morning, I visited with the marketing director of another facility. She gave me a tour and told me about their facilities and care programs. They had a campus composed of five buildings, each a separate "community." All patients were free to wander the campus except for those in the dementia building, which was a lockdown facility. All three meals were served in the building to which the patient was assigned, and it looked like a good arrangement. All patients had help getting up and dressing each morning. Many just sat in the living room all day and watched TV, but the facility offered activities for all who would take part. They also took dementia patients through to death. They had three staff people per twenty patients—a ratio of about one to seven.

All in all, my impression was that this option was a good assisted-living facility but somehow not quite the level I expected to find for Birdie.

Other Nursing Homes

Along with all the appointments I had going on, I did some unannounced stop-in visits at other nursing homes just to walk the halls and see whatever I saw. What I saw was enough to make me sure that what I was looking for was not a regular kind of nursing home but rather a specialized assisted-living facility with an Alzheimer's unit offering special care to those with dementia.

Option 5

My next appointment was at a pleasant appearing campus with two buildings—one a two-story building that looked like a big house and the other a one-story cottage type structure. It turned out that the two-story was for regular assisted living and the cottage building contained twenty private rooms with private baths for Alzheimer's patients. My appointment was with the administrator of both facilities.

When the administrator took me into the Alzheimer's building, I was amazed at how good it smelled and how homey it felt! The room we entered was a large all-purpose room with tables for eating meals and a living room type area for group togetherness. The kitchen was right next to the tables, and the smell of the food cooking gave the place an appealing odor. As we toured the patient room areas, I was further pleased to find that there were no "nursing home smells" noticeable. I asked the administrator how they did it. Her answer was, "We work hard at it."

I also noted the attitude of the attendants and the way they were relating to the patients. When I asked about that, she told me about the Christian gentleman who owned several assisted-living facilities and his desires that Christian love be practiced in the care of all patients. And she said they had ministers come each week for worship services and a full-time activities director. There seemed to be a sincere desire to make the facility as much like home as possible for the patients. She was speaking my language! And with my strong Christian background, along with the good smells and the friendly staff, I was thinking this could be it! Then she showed me the room that would be available for Birdie—a room at the end of a short hallway. It had a nice big window with a good view, a good layout, and a nice bathroom.

As she and I talked, I found out that the other criteria I had in mind were also satisfied, including that they would take Birdie through to death.

So before I left that day, we agreed that the administrator would put a hold on that room until I had a chance to talk with my family at a Thanksgiving get-together I was planning. (It was already mid-November when I visited this facility). I left just praising the Lord for finally finding a place that I felt would suit Birdie's needs with Christian love!

If God brings you to it
He will bring you through it!

—Unknown

Chapter 9

Family Decision Time

As I searched for the right care facility for Birdie, a lot of thoughts about the next steps ran through my head: *What will the family say? Will they accept my research and thinking on the matter of placing their mom in an assisted-living facility? Will they say it is too soon? Or will they have other ideas about how we should face the future as it unfolds?*

With that in mind, the more immediate question for me was how I would get all four sons and their wives together at the same time so that the nine of us could resolve this issue. The solution was to invite all the family to come to our house for a big Thanksgiving dinner. The invitations went out and contained the words "Probably the last Thanksgiving dinner in this house, and to honor Birdie for all she means to us."

Twenty-three family members came for Thanksgiving dinner! We set up a big long table from the dining room into the living room so that we were all at one table. My daughter-in-law Karen was in charge of the dinner. In its preparation, she was assisted by the other three daughters-in-law, Pam, Cindy, and Lindsey. What a feast we enjoyed together that day.

As part of our festivities, I gave a toast to Birdie that went something like this: "Let's all give a toast to honor Birdie. Without her, none of us would be here! If it were not for her, I would not be here today. And none of our four sons would be here—or their four wives. And without the daughters-in-law, there would be no grandchildren here today. And without the grandchildren, we would not have our first great-grandchild here today. So our toast to Birdie is that without her, none of us would be here today. And what a job she has done as wife, mother, mother-in-law, grandmother, and now a great-grandmother. Let's all say a big thanks to her for all she has done for us and for making this happy occasion today possible!"

Birdie was doing fairly good that day, and I think she understood at least part of what we were saying. It is hard to say what she made of it, but at least she had a big smile for us that day.

After the dinner table was cleared, the four sons, four daughters-in-law, and I went to our lower-level walk-out area of the house, where we could talk in private about the issue at hand. I presented a written paper outlining the research I had done, how the caregiving responsibilities were starting to wear on me, and my feeling that the time had come for Birdie to have professional full-time care—both for her sake as well as mine. I reviewed all the financial aspects of how the big nursing home bills would be paid, how the admittance would be handled, and so on.

Following several questions and more discussion, all nine of us agreed that the time had come. We agreed on my recommendation of the option 5 assisted-living facility, and we set the date for after Christmas with the admission date I had suggested of January 16, 2007.

Now the question was how I felt about it once the decision had been made. I had quite a mixture of feelings about what had come up in our discussions:

a. One of the reasons for approval had been the family's observation that I was looking haggard and worn-out. I knew I felt that way but had not realized how much it was apparent to others in the way I looked.

b. The finality of it was difficult. Yes, I knew that Alzheimer's was a slow downhill disease and that this day had to come eventually, but it is still a very hard decision for a husband to make. I realized she was leaving home for the last time!

c. I was glad to have all the family in agreement and that all had taken part in the decision. What a big help it was to have them check my thinking and, in the end, say, "Yes, we must proceed."

d. I was concerned about facing the day of admittance. If she was having a "good day," it could be traumatic, and she could object to the whole thing. So it was agreed that my son Mark would take that morning off from his doctor duties to accompany me in the admittance process. That decision helped allay my fears of what that day might be like.

e. All in all, I was glad that the session was over, that it went so well, and that I was ready to proceed with the remaining one and a half months of caregiving.

Cast all your anxiety on Him
because He cares for you!

—1 Peter 5:7

Chapter 10

Frustrations of a Caregiver

One of the big frustrations I encountered as a caregiver was dealing with the ups and downs of dementia.

One day would be a very down day for my wife, and I would feel that I might have waited too long in the decisions to move her to an assisted-living facility. I felt that the conditions were getting beyond my capabilities and that she was beyond the staying-at-home stage.

Then in the very same week, she would have a lucid day. At that point I wondered what in the world I had been thinking when I'd thought that she was entering the severe stage of Alzheimer's disease. That good day she could form sentences, was up most of the day, ate well, and talked about going shopping. Wow! Was it all my imagination that she needed assisted living? I wondered.

So I looked up more references on the Internet and found other caregivers saying it is normal to question the diagnosis when your loved one has moments of lucidity. The best advice I found was to enjoy the lucid moments and realize that these moments might last for a few minutes or sometimes for a couple of hours or more. But then the lucid moments are all gone, leaving you back in the reality of the situation.

Reading items like this on the Internet was very helpful to me, since this was my first time through the process of serving as a caregiver to a person with dementia. I knew that her memory was very poor, that she had trouble with activities that had once been familiar, that she had great difficulty in trying to find the words to express herself, that she had incontinence, that she could no longer dress herself, that she could not get out of a chair by herself, that I had to constantly watch to keep her from falling again, that she could not find food by herself, that I had to take care of all her pills and do all the housework, that she did not know what day it was or what time it was, and so on. But when those lucid moments came along, it seemed that the long list of her inabilities was all in my imagination.

And then tomorrow would come, the disease was again in control, and I felt frustrated with the ups and downs as each day went by.

I guess I was afraid that maybe I was proceeding too fast in my plans to place her in an assisted-living facility within the next month. Most days I felt that the time had come. Some days I felt that the move was past due. But then the lucid day would come, and I would say, "Donald, what is your rush?" Add to that the frustration of that fact that when we attended family gatherings, she usually rallied for the occasion.

Then I felt like it appeared to the family that I was exaggerating her downhill slide.

But part of the reasoning for moving my wife to assisted living was my own physical and mental health. I was bored staying at home all the time as a babysitter. I felt isolated in giving up all my social activities and felt hopeless in seeing the disease slowly take her downhill. It was starting to wear on me, and then I would think of what I had seen the caregiving role do to others, many of whom aged very rapidly in the role I was fulfilling. So was I being selfish in thinking of myself, or did God have bigger things in mind for me, especially when trained people were willing and able to take over my caregiving roles?

On her better days, Birdie occasionally expressed feelings of loneliness and her desire to be with people. When those expressions came, I again felt that I was on the right track, in that assisted living would give her companionship with other ladies who were facing the same problems with dementia.

After having had three outside professionals give their appraisals of my wife's situation, and all of them saying that she was entering the severe stage of Alzheimer's, I felt confident that I was on the right track, that the Lord had helped me find the right place for her, that the Lord had provided a staff that took a Christian approach to caring, that the family had agreed in backing me up on my decisions, that her physician had signed the long-term care insurance papers, that the assisted-living facility's evaluation was consistent with the others, and that I had mentioned the coming need for assisted living to Birdie many times.

So what were my fears? I think the biggest was that I was giving up too soon, that I should continue on for a longer period of time, that she might not be as bad as I thought she was (especially on the more lucid days), and that I was being selfish in thinking of my own well-being.

On the other hand, if the roles were reversed, and I was the one with the dementia, then I would want her to go ahead and find the best place possible for me. I wouldn't want her to go downhill taking care of me. I would hope that she could go on with her life but that she would still care for me, visit me, and see that I was properly taken care of. Those were the things I planned to do.

Maybe my biggest fear was simply what would happen the day of the move. How would she handle it? How would I handle it? It would be somewhat like a final good-bye for me, but for her, with her mind not working most of the time, it might be far easier than I imagined. All I could do was place it in the Lord's hands, pray for His continued guidance and aid, and trust in Him to see me through this rough assignment. I told myself how He had moved many mountains before, and I was sure that He had more than enough power to move this one also!

Perhaps the words of Rabbi Hillel, one of the great sages of Judaism, are most appropriate here: "If I am not for myself, who will be? If I am only for myself, what am I? And, if not now, when?" He was a wise man, and he recognized the need for all of us to have balance in our lives and to serve ourselves as well as others. His message is a wake-up call to all of us, especially to family caregivers like me, that loving yourself is not selfish. It is in fact a way of honoring and valuing the wonder of human life.

The truth is that a person can easily lose his or her true identity while being a caregiver to a spouse with dementia. You can no longer talk things over with your husband or wife, you know that the future of the disease has no hope for recovery, and you realize that the best you can do is make his or her days as comfortable as possible. Without any hope of recovery, and only more problems day by day, the task often seems dauntless! The solution for me was to spend time in prayer, asking God for his guidance day by day and trusting in His wisdom to know what to do next!

I, the Lord, your God
Will uphold your right hand,
Saying to you,
"I will help you!"

—Isaiah 41:10

Chapter 11

Worries about Admittance Day

After the family decision was made, the next task was to go through all the preparatory phases for the day when the actual move to the assisted-living facility would occur. There were many forms to be completed, such as medical and personal information forms for the assisted-living facility and forms from Birdie's doctor for the long-term care insurance coverage payments. Additional planning included determining what personal items, pictures, and furniture we would place in Birdie's room to make it seem more like home, thinking about the clothing she would need, gathering prescription information, and the like. But over and beyond all of that were my continuing concerns about whether this was the right thing to do and what would happen on the day of actual admittance.

I was so glad that my son Mark had agreed to plan ahead so that he could be available that morning to help us make the move. Birdie was continuing the slow downhill slide, but she did have better days occasionally, and I was worried that if she had a good day on the day of the move, she might raise a fuss about being left in a strange place.

The administrator had helped my worries somewhat when she told me, "If that happens, then the best thing is for you and Mark to simply walk away, leave the building, and let us take care of the situation. Birdie will not be the first case we have had where something like this happens. Usually such patients settle down after a half hour or less and in fact forget all about what the fuss was about." This information was helpful to me, and yet the heavy thoughts to me were, *This is my wife that I am doing this to!* and *Is this the right thing to do?*

In times like this, where do I turn? With my strong Christian faith, the natural thinking was to turn to the Bible. And what did I find there? Well, no direct answers to my worries ... or did I? The Bible is full of scriptures on putting your faith in God, of not worrying about tomorrow, of assurances that God cares for me and Birdie, of praising God for all the previous victories in the many struggles of life, and of facing the future with confidence. Here are just a few helpful scriptures:

- Mathew 6:34: Jesus says, "Take no worry about tomorrow—each day has enough trouble of his own."
- Philippians 4:6–7: "Do not be anxious about anything, but in everything, by prayer and petition, with thanksgiving, present your requests to God. And the peace of God, which

transcends all understanding, will guard your hearts and minds in Christ Jesus."

- Proverbs 20:24: "A man's steps are commanded by the Lord, how then can anyone understand his own way?"

Along with Bible study and prayer, I read many more caregiving articles and books on how other people had handled and conquered these worries. I also came to the realization that most of the patients in the full nursing homes I had visited were loved by families that had gone through these same concerns and worries. Good Christian hymns were a blessing at this time, as tunes would come to mind like "Leaning on the Everlasting Arms," which includes a verse that says, "What have I to dread, what have I to fear, leaning on the Everlasting Arms, I have blessed peace with my Lord so near, leaning on the Everlasting Arms!" A great help!

The month and a half between "decision day" to admittance day went by fairly quickly. Christmas came and went, and the stacks of paperwork for the admittance were completed.

Then, on the Sunday before the Tuesday of planned admittance, everything changed!

Around noon on Sunday, January 14, 2007, Birdie and I were finishing lunch on our stools at the kitchen counter. She slipped and fell to the floor as she was getting off her stool. She was crying out in pain! I tried to help her but realized it might be serious and that I had better call for help. Luckily, my doctor son Mark, who lived down the street, had just gotten home from church. He rushed to our house, did his examination, and said he thought she had broken her hip! We called the ambulance and had her rushed to the hospital.

The diagnosis was a broken hip. Hip replacement surgery was scheduled for the following evening. The surgery went well, but she developed some problems and was kept in the hospital for ten days.

The hospital stated that she needed to be placed in a nursing home for rehabilitation. I did not want to see this happen for fear that she never would get out. I talked with the assisted-living facility, and they agreed to take her directly from the hospital and said they could give her all the physical care she needed. The hospital finally agreed to this plan.

Now I really had mixed feelings! On one hand, all my worries about the day of admittance had been resolved. Was this the way God had answered my prayers? He made it so much easier for me and maybe for Birdie also. But on the other hand, why did Birdie have to go through the misery of a broken hip on top of all the other problems of recent years? Whatever the answers to those questions were, at least the answers on how to handle admission day were now in place.

What were Birdie's reactions to the broken hip? It was hard to say. Her mind was not with it enough to fully comprehend what had happened, yet she seemed to know it was not good. She groaned with pain but settled down as the ambulance and hospital personnel took over in giving her pain relief and excellent care in the situation at hand. The ambulance transfer from the hospital to the assisted-living facility went smoothly. The big move from home to assisted living was now complete!

I lift my eyes to the mountains---
Where does my help come from?
My help comes from the Lord,
The maker of heaven and earth!

—Psalm 121:1–2

Chapter 12

Assisted-Living Situations

Birdie was in the assisted-living facility for eighteen months, from January 2007 to July 2008. During those months, I was very pleased with the loving care she received. Her room was kept clean and cheery, she was neatly dressed, each day she received excellent personal care, the food was very good, the prescriptions were properly administered, and I was welcomed when I went for daily visits.

I found that going in the morning was usually not good, since that was when the staff members were getting her going for the day (breakfast, cleaning, dressing, etc.) plus there was usually a morning activity of some kind. Sometimes I would go around ten thirty in the morning and join in the group activity (or sit and watch) and then leave when lunch was ready. (I could stay for meals with the group if I reserved in advance.) My usual time was to go around midafternoon, after her afternoon nap, when I could join in the afternoon activity or we could just sit in her room and watch TV. If I had reserved in advance, I would stay for dinner;

they would seat me at one of the tables next to Birdie and some of the patients would attempt conversation.

But overall, I found it best to time my visits so that I was leaving when she was ready for an activity, such as dinnertime. This seemed to relieve the problem I encountered during the early months of how to answer her pleas of "Don't leave me here," "I want to go home with you," or simply "I want to be with you!" How do you respond to requests like that? The answer that seemed to work best was to say, "The doctor says you are not ready yet." That seemed to satisfy her somewhat, but I still found it very hard to leave my wife of more than fifty years when she was begging to go with me.

As the first month went by, I found it to be a very common thing for Alzheimer's patients to say what Birdie was saying to me: "Don't leave me here," etcetera. I heard other patients saying the same things to their families.

Then one afternoon when Birdie was having a good day, I offered to take her for a ride. Using one of the available wheelchairs, I got her out of the facility and into the car. She seemed to really enjoy the ride. After about a half hour or so, she told me, "I'm feeling tired. I want to go home." Well, at first I thought "home" meant our home, but then I realized that apparently she was talking about her room at the assisted-living facility. So I got her back to her room, and she seemed glad to be "home." From then on I felt better about what home meant to her.

There were some happier occasions provided by the assisted-living facility, including events to which I was invited and a few to which our family was invited. One such event was a musical program with a pianist and vocal soloist. Another was a Christmas party with Santa Claus. I attended a few of their Sunday morning worship services with guest ministers. They also had storytellers and other similar events. These events provided opportunities for the patients to have their families visit with something for the family to do. I'm not sure how much the patients got from the programs (maybe more than I think!), but it seemed to bring them joy in having their loved ones in for the evening. I was pleased with the efforts made to make the place feel like home for the patients.

For Birdie's eightieth birthday, we were allowed to use the boardroom for a family luncheon to celebrate the occasion. We had carry-in dinners, flowers, a big birthday cake, and so forth. Birdie seemed to enjoy the occasion, but I am not sure she understood what it was all about.

We celebrated two wedding anniversaries during her time there—our fifty-second and fifty-third. For these, the activities director planned and served a very special first-class luncheon to Birdie and me in her room. She set up a small table with two chairs, a table cloth, flowers, a fancy meal, and a cake. This, I thought, was very special care!

One day when I went to visit, Birdie told me that some nice young man came to see her. She did not know who it was. I mentioned some names, but none seemed to ring a bell with her. So I went out to see the guest registry. Guess who had come. Our son Mark! That was the first occasion of her not recognizing her own family members. Later, she did not seem to know me, except that I was the guy who came to visit her regularly.

One blessing of Alzheimer's disease is that as the memory fails, worries disappear. Birdie no longer had the paranoia of people plotting against her, and she no longer worried about family problems. In that respect, it appears that from the patient's point of view, the final months are not all that bad. It may be that the caregiver is the one who suffers most during the final months.

During Birdie's eighteen months at the assisted-living facility, she had at least four different hospital stays of varying lengths. She fell in June 2007, breaking her pelvis. In August 2007 she fell again, breaking her other hip. Then in February 2008, I received a phone call at 1:40 a.m. stating that Birdie had been taken to the hospital, this time diagnosed with edema.

By the time I got there, they had utilized the full emergency team and there were tubes going down her nose and throat to try to get the fluid out of her lungs. As the rush settled down, I talked with the emergency room doctor about the living will in Birdie's medical files, which the assisted-living facility had given to the ambulance driver. In the living will, she had requested that no big emergency procedures be used if something like this should happen.

The doctor explained to me that their first concern was to do whatever they could to save the life of the patient and worry about reading the patient's files later. (I found this to be true with other patients' experiences.) I talked with the assisted-living administrator about this and asked why they had even sent Birdie to the hospital when the living will said to take no heroic measures. Her answer was that according to their licensing, they were required to send a patient to the hospital whenever the patient's needs were beyond their facilities (they did not have RNs on staff twenty-four hours per day). Birdie recovered from this incident and was released back to the assisted-living facility. On July 8, 2008, she was again rushed to the hospital, this time with pneumonia, and the same emergency procedures were employed. On July 12, she was released back to the assisted-living facility and placed on hospice. She died four days later, on July 18, 2008.

After being placed on hospice, Birdie seemed much more relaxed. She was no longer forced to take medicines, did not have to eat if she did not want to, and could have all the morphine she wanted to control any pain. For her, the last few days of life seemed much easier, and for that I was grateful. She had suffered enough!

Whatever is true, whatever is noble,
whatever is right, whatever is pure,
whatever is lovely, whatever is admirable,
---if anything is excellent or praiseworthy---
THINK ABOUT SUCH THINGS!

—Philippians 4:8

Chapter 13

Notes to Myself

Who do you talk to when you come home after a bad day visiting your loved one? The house is empty. Your spouse is gone. You feel like you need to unload to someone.

I found that sitting down at the computer and simply writing a note to myself seemed to get it off my chest, and I found it helpful to go back after several days had passed and see how I had felt on those low days. The following are a few examples of such notes to myself. You will note changes that occurred between the first two and the last two.

July 18, 2007
Today seemed especially hard.

Birdie wants me to do a favor for her: she wants to go to our house.

They are not treating her good. They want her to do everything their way.

She doesn't want to stay there any longer.

She was cold. I put sweater on her and then added a blanket.

Had a good chat with her caregiver. She says that Birdie is doing better. She's eating again and sleeping better again. She thinks Birdie is starting to recover from her fractured pelvis and from the intense pain of the fracture.

Birdie did not want me to leave. She wanted me to stay with her.

Her mind seemed fairly good compared to the others there today, but she had trouble finding the words. She couldn't remember anything short-term.

I'm getting used to the constant requests to go home. That is part of the disease. But it is still hard, especially on days when her mind is fairly clear.

All in all, the downhill slide continues, some days more than others. She has been there six months now. I could no longer take care of her at home.

But it is still hard—the guilt feelings, the firmness I have to use when I leave, seeing her so sad to see me go, and so on.

Lord, what are the answers?

July 19, 2007

Lin (my daughter-in-law Lindsey) went with me this evening to try suits on Birdie for her granddaughter's wedding, which was coming up soon.

Birdie was still in great pain from her fractured pelvis. We tried one jacket on her, but she was in too much pain to try the slacks.

When we first arrived, Birdie's first words to me were "take me home." When we were ready to leave, she again pleaded, "Don't leave me."

It is hard. And it is getting to the point where perhaps I seem harsh with her.

My reactions were as follows:

1. Maybe she is reverting to second childhood.
2. Maybe she is becoming more "clingy" again.
3. I should listen to the administrator's advice to skip visiting for a few days, that I am coming to visit more for my sake than for hers.
4. Perhaps she does get along better when I do not show up. She seems to look at me to solve her problems.
5. Lindsey agrees that I should skip days.

Lord, help me! What is the correct way to go? I am providing for her the best help available, much better than I can do. In fact, she is now way beyond what I could take care of.

April 3, 2008
Birdie was very quiet today.

We joined group at table for coffee and cookies. She partook but said nothing.

Later she had frown on her face. I tried to see what was wrong, whether she had to go to the bathroom or had pains. She said she had pain but did not know where. Then she said, "Leave me alone!"

That's the first I have heard her say that for a long time!

I talked with an attendant. She says Birdie has been having spells like this for the past few days. I'm not sure what is wrong. A new phase of the disease?

Of the six ladies at the table today for coffee and cookies, Birdie was the quietest. Others opened up and talked fairly well about their younger lives.

So what goes?

My opinion is she is getting weaker. Her mind is closing down more. Where does it all go? Three more months? Six more months? Or years?

Only the Lord knows! And He is in control. And Birdie's faith in Him has remained very strong!

April 9, 2008

Went to visit Birdie today at 3:15 p.m. She was at church service in the building. I went there to join the group.

She seemed kind of dazed today. She had a bland, far-off look in the eyes and did not seem to know who I was. She was breathing hard and had that painful-looking frown on her face.

My thoughts were, *How much longer can she last?*

Then I realized that she is already way beyond what I thought it would be. A year ago I did not think she would make it to the spring of 2008!

When I talk to her and say, "The Lord is good," she smiles and says something like, "He sure is!" So I believe her faith is still very strong. Praise the Lord!

Today she did not object when I left. She just asked, "When are you coming back?"

So I left feeling both helpless and frustrated, but I was also glad that I was able to arrange such good and caring help for her. She is being well taken care of!

These few examples of notes to myself may be an idea you can use to help clarify your thoughts as you care for your loved one. It was helpful to me. Even now, after several years have passed, it is revealing to me to relive some of the feelings I went through in those trying days.

One of the questions you probably noted that I dealt with was, *How long does this go on?*

From what I have read and studied on this topic, plus my experience watching various patients in the assisted-living facility, it would appear that Birdie's case was about average. I observed many who went faster and also some who went very slowly. At least two of the patients were there before Birdie was admitted and did not die until several months after Birdie was gone. On the other hand, I observed many who came in after Birdie did and were gone before Birdie was. So, like any other illness, it all depends. Some go fast, some go slow.

Another good point in the above notes was the advice to skip some days. This I started to do, and it seemed to help the situation. It was probably harder for me to stay away than it was for Birdie not to see me, and it saved her all the parting problems when I would leave. It also helped that I always knew she was being well cared for.

I have learned to be content
Whatever the circumstances

—Apostle Paul (Phil. 4:11)

Chapter 14

How to Maintain a Positive Attitude While My Wife Is Going Downhill

One of the big challenges I faced—and you will face—is keeping your attitude on the positive side as caregiving tasks grow more wearisome each day. I often wondered, *How can I possibly keep my mind on positive thoughts while my wife is going downhill? She has been my sounding board for the past fifty years, as I have been for her. But now our communications are next to nil. Her mind has gone to a different world. I miss our chats together. I am still here to take care of her body. How in the world do I keep myself from becoming distressed? At the same time, I recognize that it is a must that I keep myself upbeat if I am to be able to continue in the many daily tasks involved in being a loving caregiver. So it is not only for my own sake but more so for the sake of my failing wife that I must work at the task of keeping on going on! Where do I turn for help?*

In my first book, *FORWARD EVER*, I listed some of the keys I'd found to maintaining a positive attitude during the years of job pressures, time pressures, family problems, and all those things we endure during our younger years of life. The good news is that I have found that those same keys also work during our senior years, including the years in the role as caregiver. The following are some of those keys.

First and foremost for me is the Christian faith. The Bible offers so much advice in how to make life decisions—especially in how we should look at ourselves and others, and how we relate to our creator. Here are a few of the Bible verses I memorized and thought about often:

Christ gives us the real challenge in Mathew 17:20, where he tells us, "If you have faith as small as a grain of mustard seed, you can say to this mountain 'move from here to there' and it will move. Nothing will be impossible to you!" This is a verse I pondered for years. As a child I thought about actual mountains of earth being moved. But as years went by, I realized that God was moving mountains for me—mountains of doubt, fear, and problems that were beyond my abilities to solve. What an awesome God we serve! And yes, He does move mountains!

Paul gives us another challenge for mind control in Philippians 4:8, where he tells us, "Finally, brothers, whatever is pure, whatever is lovely, whatever is admirable—if anything is excellent or praise-worthy—*think about such things.*" These words from Paul have been very helpful to me in emphasizing that what we put into our minds has so much to do with the words and actions that come out of us. When I am involved in a bad or difficult situation, I think of this scripture and realize that there are also many good things going on around me that I could think about. Then I purposely choose to see if I can concentrate on those things. It is not easy, but it is a choice that you and I can make, and it is certainly worth the effort!

And further on in the same chapter, Paul says in Philippians 4:11, "I have learned to be content whatever the circumstances—through Him who gives me the strength." Wow! What an achievement in faith to arrive at that stage of controlling your own mind, thoughts, and attitude! If Paul could do that after all he suffered through, why can't you and I strive for that same level of contentment in Christ?

Proverbs 23:7 sums it up quite well: "As a man thinketh, so is he."

Another source of inspiration for me was to look at the wall in my office, where I have a bronze plaque with the words of the Optimist Creed—a creed I learned and repeated each week during my twenty-five years as a member of Optimist International. I served as president of the club in Anderson, Indiana, and later as lieutenant governor in the state of Indiana. This creed contains so many good thoughts on controlling your mind, so much so that I want to share it with you here for your consideration:

The Optimist Creed

Promise yourself:

To be so strong that nothing can disturb your peace of mind.

To talk health, happiness, and prosperity to every person you meet.

To make all your friends feel that there is something in them.

To look at the sunny side of everything and make your optimism come true.

To think only of the best, to work only for the best, and to expect only the best.

To be just as enthusiastic about the success of others as you are about your own.

To forget the mistakes of the past and press on to the achievements of the future.

To wear a cheerful countenance at all times and give every living creature you meet a smile.

To give so much time to the improvement of yourself that you have no time to criticize others.

To be too large for worry, too noble for anger, too strong for fear, and too happy to permit the presence of trouble!

—*Optimist International*

If you find the above helpful, you also might want to read a book I read a number of years ago: *Learned Optimism* by Martin Seligman. This book gives many tips and examples of people who have successfully used the power of positive thinking to make their lives more enjoyable. It could work for you, despite whatever circumstances you may find yourself in, including the role of being a caregiver.

Often my mind would be calmed by letting the words of a familiar hymn run through the background of my thoughts. Here are a few examples of the type of tunes that helped me through many days.

"Leaning on the Everlasting Arms" is based on the scripture in Deuteronomy 33:27: "the Eternal God is thy refuge, and underneath are the everlasting arms." On days when I felt like I needed to lean on something bigger than myself, the words of the refrain of that song ran through my head over and over: "Leaning, leaning, safe and secure from all alarms. Leaning, leaning, leaning on the everlasting arms."

And I would remember some of the words of the three verses:

Verse 1
What a fellowship, what a joy divine,
Leaning on the everlasting arms.
What a blessedness, what a peace is mine,
Leaning on the everlasting arms.

Verse 2
O how sweet to walk in the pilgrim way,
Leaning on the everlasting arms.
O how bright the path, grows from day to day,
Leaning on the everlasting arms.

Verse 3
What have I to dread, what have I to fear,
Leaning on the everlasting arms.
I have blessed peace, with my Lord so near,
Leaning on the everlasting arms.

A second helpful tune was "Because He Lives, I Can Face Tomorrow," written by Bill Gaither. Here are the powerful words of this good tune that will fill your mind with hope:

Because he lives, I can face tomorrow.
Because He lives, all fear is gone.
Because I know He holds the future
And life is worth the living, just because
He lives!

The words of a couple of the verses of this song can also help to review and renew your faith and remind you that this life is not the end:

Verse 1
God sent his Son, they called him Jesus.
He came to love, heal, and forgive.
He lived and dies to buy my pardon.
An empty grave is there to prove my Savior lives.

Verse 2
And then one day, I'll cross the river.
I'll fight life's final war with pain.
And then, as death gives way to victory,
I'll see the lights of glory, and I'll know He
lives.

One more hymn has words of encouragement that helped me and might help you in the struggles you are now facing. This hymn was written by Charles A. Tindley and is titled "We Will Understand It Better By and By." The chorus has these great words for looking to the future:

We will understand it better by and by.
When the morning comes,
When the saints of God are gathered home,
We'll tell the story how we've overcome.
We will understand it better by and by!

This hymn is based on the words of Paul as found in 1 Corinthians 13:12. He says, "Now we see but a poor reflection: then we shall see face to face. Now I know in part, then I shall know fully even as I am fully known." In other words, we don't have all the answers now, but someday we will be able to see and talk with Christ and then we will comprehend! I am looking forward to that day!

The verses of this hymn say it very well:

Verse 1
Trials dark on every hand, and we cannot understand
All the ways that God would lead us to that Promised Land,
But he will guide us with his eye and we will follow 'til we die.

Verse 2
When our cherished plans have failed,
Disappointments have prevailed,
And we've wandered in the darkness, heavy hearted and alone,
But we are trusting in the Lord and according to his word.

Verse 3
Temptations, hidden snares, often take us unawares,
And our hearts are made to bleed
For some thoughtless word or deed,
And we wonder why the test, when we try to do our best.

None of the above will necessarily change any of the problems you now face, but you will see the problems differently and find new solutions to the problems of the day as your mind explores new options in a positive way. Negative thinking, on the other hand, closes doors of opportunity so that the hole you are in just gets deeper and deeper.

In my college psychology classes, one of the assigned books was by Hans Selye. It was titled *Stress without Distress*. Here is an excerpt from that book that applies to all stages of life, including life as a caregiver:

> Try to keep your mind constantly on the pleasant aspects of life, and on the actions you can take to improve your situation. Try to forget everything that is irrevocably ugly or painful. This is perhaps the most efficient way of minimizing stress by what I have called voluntary mental diversion. As a wise German proverb says, "imitate the sundial's ways, count only the pleasant days."

In that same vein, another help to me was to change my evening prayers from "gimme" prayers to "thank you" prayers by thinking of only the good things that happened that day. The prayer style that developed for me was to think of all the events of the day in sequence and in doing so come up with twenty-five good things for which to say thanks. As I go through the day, bad things also come to mind, but I tell the Lord, "I'll come back to that later. Right now all I want to do is praise You for all the good things of this day." It is amazing how many good things happened—needs supplied, little successes, phone calls, helpful scriptures, sunshine, shelter. All kinds of good things will come to your mind. The big blessing is that many times before I finish the list, I fall asleep for the night. What a blessed way to fall asleep: counting your blessings.

My last bit of advice for this chapter is an adage you have heard many times: "Live in day-tight compartments." I found this short little sentence of help on many days, days when I found myself worrying about tomorrow or next week or next month and wondered how in the world I could ever handle all the problems I could see coming my way. Then I would ask myself, "Can I handle today's problems?" And then I would give the answer to that question: "Yes, I can!" This simple question may be of help to you like it was to me. Or as the Bible says, "Today's problems are sufficient unto themselves."

Do not withhold good
From those who deserve it
'When it is in your power
To help them!

—Proverbs 3:27

Chapter 15

How Do I Pray for My Wife?

I am a believer in the power of prayer. God has answered so many prayers for me during this journey of life—prayers in difficult situations, in illness of loved ones or myself, in fact, in all kinds of life situations. But how do you or I pray for our spouses when they are going downhill with Alzheimer's?

I have seen some miraculous healings, but no where in my knowledge have there been any cases of the reversal of advanced Alzheimer's disease. So my faith for healing does not seem to be well-founded in this case.

In many ways, the grief process is already underway at that stage. Your loved one's mind is nearly gone, but the body remains. What sense does it make to keep the body going when your husband or wife has already departed that body and it is only an empty shell? Yes, the living body being there does remind you daily of all the good years you had together, but those days are gone.

So my prayers changed from prayers for healing to prayers for the "eternal healing," the completion of this life cycle, to relieve my wife of the struggles she fought against so bravely and, on the selfish side, to relieve me of the caregiving role I had been in for so long. The problem for me was that such prayer sounded so selfish on my part. Yes, I was tired of the caregiving routine for a physical body that my wife used to live in.

A book I found quite helpful at that time was *God Never Forgets—Faith Hope, and Alzheimer's Disease*, edited by Donald K. McKim and published by Westminster Press. Here is an excerpt from that book:

> The ravages of the disease force us to reconsider, too, the concept heroic suffering, especially for the caregiver. As psychologist Judah Rouch argues, long term, progressive illness like Alzheimer's prevents the patient and caregiver from coming to terms with dying as a process within the life cycle. There is no chance for consolidation or saying goodbye in this process. *Survivors must grieve the separation from and the loss of all that was the person while the person is still physically present to trigger memories of what is lost.* Roles change as the spouse moves from being lover to caregiver, spouseless but married.
>
> An Alzheimer's spouses described this process as *"Death would be better than*

this –to hold on to the box when the present is used up—hoping the box can bring again the joy of the reality of the gift—but the box is empty!" This is what one has to look forward to with Alzheimer's disease.

On another page in this same book, we find the following:

> God is with Alzheimer's caregivers, unconditionally, as they struggle with their loss of dreams for the future and their feelings of anger, frustration, loneliness, confusion, jealousy, depression, and envy. Caregivers also suffer under the heroic and judgmental expectations about suffering in the Bible. Instead, a "good enough solution" ought to be the central task of caregiving.

Or, as a book on caregiving strategies recommends:

> Too often, caregivers evaluate their efforts against unrealistic standards ... Sometimes, despite the well thought out, best efforts of caregivers, persons with Alzheimer's will still react in troubling, painful ways, that they are somehow inadequate, that "if only" they were better or different, the outbursts

would never occur. *Are you dooming yourself to feeling constantly inadequate because you unconsciously think: If I do everything right then she will never have an outburst"? If so, it is time to reevaluate the yardstick by which you judge.*

Certainly God accepts us as we are and doesn't demand this kind of heroic and virtuous perfection.

Here is one more excerpt that spoke to me about the subject of how to pray for my wife at this stage of the disease.

When spouses become caregivers for their cognitively impaired spouse, they remember the part of the *marriage vow "to love and cherish in sickness and in health, "til death do us part."* The critical concern in this context may be the quality of life for the spouse who does not have Alzheimer's disease. Often the world of the caregiving spouse shrinks to the geography of the house and maybe the grocery store. Friends tend to stay away, and the caregiver is alone 24 hours of the day with a spouse in the advanced stages of the disease often no longer knows the caregiver. The quality of life for this caregiving person becomes marginal at best.

Reading passages like these was helpful in relieving my feelings of being selfish for praying to God that this ordeal might soon be over, for her sake and mine. I felt that she had suffered long enough. Any hope of recovery short of a big miracle was very slim, and this ordeal was wearing me down. If your spouse is getting into the final stages of the disease, my guess is that you are starting to feel the same way. For those of us who are Christians, our belief in Christ's promise of the better life that follows this one makes us desire for our spouses to escape this misery and precede us in celebrating the new life where such afflictions are no more!

He put a new song in my mouth
A hymn of praise to our God!

—Psalm 40:3

Chapter 16

Caregiving Days Are Over. Now What?

You have spent the past several or many years as a caregiver. Now your spouse has died. You have held the funeral. The family has gone home. You sit down in your easy chair and say, "Now what?"

You are now entering a new stage of your life. What kind of life do you want it to be? Are there things you have always wanted to do? Do you have a prioritized bucket list? Do you want to get married again? Do you want to change your living situation? Move to a condo? Do you have needs to get taken care of? Or maybe you just want to settle back, rest for a few months, and catch up with yourself.

I asked myself questions like this: Can I now devote more time to my church again? Do my friends remember me? Am I still welcome in our social groups? Are there volunteer jobs I would like to try? Do I want to write a book? These are just some of the possibilities that rumbled through my mind.

So what did I decide to do in this endeavor to "build a new life" without my wife of fifty-three years?

In the next couple chapters, I will tell you about a few of the things I did in this "new life" and the many adjustments involved. Some of the things I did may appeal to you or give you ideas to ponder as you decide how you want to approach this new stage in life.

May the God of all grace,
Who called us to His eternal glory
By Christ Jesus,
After you have suffered a while,
Perfect, establish, strengthen and settle you!

—1 Peter 5:10

Chapter 17

Cruise to Alaska

One of the first things that appeared on my bucket list was to go to Alaska. I had been to forty-nine of the fifty states but never to Alaska. Now was my chance. Why not go? I found a last-minute deal on Holland America for a cruise from Anchorage to Vancouver. So in early September I flew to Anchorage, took the train to Seward to board the ship, and off I went.

I took along several books on the grief process that I wanted to read, thinking that since I would be cruising by myself, I would have time to sit in a nice area and educate myself on what others had learned about facing life without the one you love. I did find some time for that, and I found it very helpful to compare myself with others who had traveled the same path.

But there were also new friends. On the first day out, the ship announced a luncheon for all singles on board. About thirty or forty singles showed up, and we enjoyed lunch together. So that gave us singles some acquaintances as we strolled the ship.

At the table I was assigned to in the main dining room for dinner each evening, there was a single lady who had just lost her husband. She was a retired nurse who lived in Florida. We had many conversations and enjoyed popcorn together during the evening movies on a couple of occasions. Later she told me that she had an extra bedroom in her condo in Florida and invited me to come use it anytime I was down that way! I never took her up on that invitation (she was not quite my type) but it opened my eyes to the fact that if I got myself "out and around," I just might meet that special someone who might tempt me to try marriage again. So the grief recovery process was already beginning. I was starting to think about what the future might hold.

So idea number one for you: Take a cruise. Change your views!

But those who hope in the Lord
Will renew their strength.
They will soar on wings like eagles:
They will run and not grow weary,
They will walk and not be faint!

—Isaiah 40:31

Chapter 18

Hospice Weekend Retreat—
Retreat, Reflect, Renew

When I returned from the Alaskan cruise, I found an invitation waiting for me to attend a weekend workshop sponsored by hospice. It was to be held at a nice retreat center in central Michigan and was for people who had recently lost loved ones. It was to begin with dinner on Friday evening and conclude with lunch on Sunday at noon. It was scheduled for late October. The invitation said,

> *This autumn, take the time you need to find your balance and foster the deep peace that can only come from gently nurturing your mind, body, and spirit.*

It sounded like just what I needed in this whole grief recovery process. So I signed up.

There were about twenty-five registrants, mostly widows and widowers who had recently lost their spouses. As usual at this age, most of the participants were ladies, with a few men like me mixed in. We all enjoyed a nice get-acquainted dinner on Friday evening and then the opening ceremony to introduce us to the agenda for the weekend.

Saturday was a full day of activities, speakers, and advice of various kinds. Here is a list of some of the areas covered:

Take Good Care of Yourself
Grief can affect your physical, emotional, spiritual, and mental health. Grieving and mourning can be overwhelming and exhausting. During this time in your life, it will be important to take good care of yourself. Remember, self-care is not selfish; it is necessary to help you survive.

Eat as Well as You Can
Your body needs nourishment now more than ever. Many people have a change in their appetite or eating habits when they are grieving. Try to eat small meals or healthy snacks throughout the day to help your energy level.

Exercise Regularly
Return to your old program or start a new one as soon as possible. Exercise releases tension and anxiety. Depression can be lightened a little by the biochemical changes brought by exercise, and you will sleep better. A daily walk is ideal for many people.

Spiritual Growth

Resume regular church attendance. Pray for others and for yourself. Read sacred and spiritual books and writings, and express your faith or lack of faith with others.

Exercise Your Mind

Learn new skills. Discuss current events or new ideas with others. Plan social activities or trips you would like to take. Take classes. Plan your future.

Consider Medication

Although medications may provide some relief, they should not be taken for the purpose of avoiding the pain of loss. Be sure your physician knows the type and frequency of all medications you use.

Rest and Sleep

Some degree of sleep disturbance is expected. However, lack of sufficient sleep may lead to mental and physical exhaustion. Speak with your physician if you are not able to sleep.

Pay Attention to Your Physical Health

A certain amount of physical change is a normal component of grief because grief assaults the body as well as the mind. Grieving is a time of high health risks. Seek medical treatment for physical symptoms if they develop.

Write a Letter to Your Husband or Wife

One of the exercises I found helpful was to go to a quiet place in the lodge and write a letter to my wife. Guidelines for the letter were given to us. Here are some of them:

- Start out with how you are feeling and how you are doing since your loved one passed away.
- Write about what you miss.
- Write about any regrets.
- What do you wish you had said or done before your loved one's death?
- Describe how you are coping. What makes you laugh or cry now?
- Close with any personal message you would like to include.
- When finished, place the letter in an envelope and pretend you have mailed it.

The last part of the exercise was to change places with the deceased who just received the letter and with your other hand compose a letter back to you.

This exercise helped me let go of some pent-up feelings—another step in the grief recovery process.

Start a Journal

It was emphasized that putting words on paper allows us to express our painful feelings rather than carrying them around inside us. We can pour our tears out in a journal anytime we feel like it. Our journals are always there to receive our thoughts and feelings. Journaling allows you to see your progress as you review what you wrote last week or last month. It shows how you have grown. Just the act of writing things down also makes you organize your thoughts and feelings, which in turn helps you to move on to new things.

Self-Appraisal "Quiet Stations"

Toward the end of the day, we were to go to three different "quiet stations," where handout sheets were available for us to self-appraise ourselves and our progress in three areas:

a. *Acceptance:* Am I finding the serenity within myself to let go of the past and move with confidence into the future?

b. *Resilience:* Do I have the ability to recover from or adjust easily to misfortune or change?

c. *Hope:* Do I live in hope with confidence to face the future? What progress have I seen in myself since my loved one's death?

Included in the windup session on Sunday morning was the opportunity to share with the group whatever you wanted about your reactions to the retreat and any help you felt it had been to you. I especially found help just in being with twenty-five other people who were also in the grief recovery process and discovering so many common elements in it, along with the many helpful sessions and meaningful tips for the future. I felt so much more confident about the future as I drove home. I felt as though I had retreated, refreshed, and renewed!

(One of the widows there did interest me. In the weeks after the retreat, I picked her up at her home on a couple of occasions to attend hospice follow-up meetings, but there was not enough "flame" there, so we drifted apart. But it broke the ice for me to have "first dates" after fifty-three years of marriage!)

The time of the singing
Of the birds
Is come!

—Song of Solomon 2:12

Chapter 19

Cruise to the Panama Canal and Meeting That Special Someone

Following the hospice retreat, I started to feel better about things. The load of the "grief process" was getting lighter, since I had traveled much of that road during the last year of the downward slide of my wife's Alzheimer's disease.

The busy season of Thanksgiving and Christmas came and went, but I was concerned about the long winter month of January and felt I had to plan something special for myself for that month. So I signed up for an Elder Hostel (now called Road Scholar) cruise to the Panama Canal, leaving Fort Lauderdale in mid-January 2009.

Most of the Elder Hostel sessions and tours I had attended had around twenty-five to thirty attendees, but this one had the smallest number allowed, just twelve. In the "get-acquainted" session the first evening on the ship, after we had all introduced ourselves, we proceeded to the dining room for our first dinner together. As luck would have it, I managed to sit by the most attractive lady in the group. From the introductions, I knew that her husband had died in 2008, the same year my wife had died. We had many more interesting conversations about many things as the cruise progressed during the following ten days.

Upon my return to Michigan, I decided to send her an e-mail to see if she got home okay. That started a chain of e-mails back and forth over the next six months, and in those e-mails I learned so much more about her and the many similarities of our backgrounds:

1. We were both married for fifty-three years.
2. We were both caregivers for the last six years of our marriages. Her husband had a stroke, while my wife had Alzheimer's disease.
3. Both of us had obtained our college degrees as adults. She had a master's degree in education, and I had a master's in business administration.
4. She taught school for twenty-nine years. I had been in Christian publishing for twenty-eight years.
5. She has three daughters. I have four sons.
6. She has eight grandchildren. I have nine.
7. She was very active in her church. I was very active in my church.
8. We were surprised to discover that we were both driving the same make and model of car: a 2008 Buick Lucerne.
9. We both enjoy traveling.

On and on went the list of similarities in our beliefs and backgrounds! And we thoroughly enjoyed talking with each other.

Then she surprised me when she wrote an e-mail saying she was planning to sign up for another Elder Hostel tour, this one starting in Seattle, Washington, and including a small ship cruise to ports in the Pungent Sound. She asked if I might be interested in that same tour. You can guess my answer: "Yes, I sure am interested!" So our first meeting after Panama in January was set for Seattle in September 2009.

We decided to meet in Seattle a day before the Elder Hostel meetings began. We spent that day walking through the city, sitting on park benches, and just talking about life. We were surprised that we had so much to talk about! During the months since we had seen each other on the Panama Canal trip, I had worked on cleaning out my house, disposed of all the furniture and "stuff," and had moved in with my son and his family until the house was sold. She had continued to live in the same home that she and her husband had prepared for their retirement home in New Jersey. Our talks included what-ifs for the future.

The following months brought more trips together, visits back and forth (me to her home in New Jersey and her to my home in Michigan), and daily phone calls and e-mails and texts. We just plain fell in love with each other!

Now for the good news.

We were married in a church wedding in August 2013, with all four of my sons and all three of her daughters present for the occasion. We were so delighted that all seven of our children seemed happy to see us find new love in our lives. We enjoyed honeymoons to Mackinac Island in Michigan and then a river cruise in Europe. We now are settled down in her home in Lavallette, New Jersey.

The message of this final chapter is there is always hope! Here Lois and I go again for a new life after years of struggle and caregiving for our mates, who we loved so dearly.

Now, may the Lord of peace Himself
Give you Peace always in every way.
The Lord be with you all!

—2 Thessalonians 3:16

Conclusion

I hope the many things I learned during my years of caregiving may give you some insights and aid as you face many of the same issues. It is not an easy road! There were many days when I thought, *This is just too much for me.*

It was for that reason that I included the last few chapters in this book, to let you see how the sun rises again after all the stress and strain of caregiving days are over.

May the Lord bless you and keep you day by day as you strive to provide the best possible care you know how to give.

www.ingramcontent.com/pod-product-compliance
Lightning Source LLC
Chambersburg PA
CBHW030805180526
45163CB00003B/1156